ADVANCED PILATES EXERCISE FOR EVERYONE 101

A book showcasing a variety of exercises suitable for people of all ages, fitness levels, weight loss and abilities, with clear instructions, illustrations, and tips for proper form and technique.

Lola Kim

Copyright © 2024 Lola Kim

All rights reserved. No part of this book be reproduced or transmitted in any form or by any means electronic, mechanical, including photocopying, recording or by any information storage and retrieval system, without any permission in writing from the author.

This book is a work of non-fiction. The views expressed are solely those of the author and don't necessarily reflect the views of the publisher, and the publisher hereby disclaims any responsibility for them.

INTRODUCTION

Welcome to the realm of physical fitness, where you can start living a stronger, healthier, and more energetic life. This book will address the fundamentals of physical health, a variety of exercises and activities, and the transformational potential of Pilates.

Being physically fit is about feeling good on the inside as much as it is about looking nice. It's about having the enthusiasm and drive to face life's obstacles head-on with assurance and zeal. This book is meant to be your reliable travel companion on your fitness adventure, regardless of your experience level or where you are in the fitness world.

In the following chapters, we will start by defining physical fitness and discussing its importance for overall health and well-being. We'll explore the benefits of exercise and physical activity, from improving cardiovascular health to enhancing mental clarity and reducing stress. Then, we'll dive into practical strategies for getting started with exercise, setting goals, and overcoming common barriers that may stand in your way.

Next, we'll explore the fundamentals of exercise, including cardiovascular exercise, strength training, and flexibility training. You'll learn about different types of exercises, how to perform them safely and effectively, and how to tailor your workouts to meet your individual needs and goals. We'll look at the various ways you may make movement part of your everyday routine in the physical activities section, from hiking and bicycling to using the stairs instead of the elevator. We'll also explore mind-body practices like Pilates and yoga, which build inner peace and mindfulness in addition to strengthening the body. Lastly, we'll delve deeper into the realm of Pilates, covering everything from its foundational theories and historical background to its useful applications in enhancing posture, flexibility, and core strength.

Whether you're new to Pilates or an experienced practitioner, you'll get insightful knowledge and motivation to improve your practice and broaden your comprehension of this game-changing physical activity. So, are you ready to embark on this journey to better health and vitality? Let's dive in and discover the joy of movement, the power of exercise, and the transformative potential of Pilates. Your body and mind will thank you for it.

Understanding Physical Fitness

The foundation of a happy and healthy existence is physical fitness. This chapter will discuss what physical fitness is, what makes it necessary, and why it is important for general health.

Definition of Physical Fitness

Physical fitness encompasses the ability to perform daily tasks with vigor and without undue fatigue. It involves a combination of various factors, including cardiovascular endurance, muscular strength, muscular endurance, flexibility, and body composition.

Achieving a condition of optimal health and functionality in the body and mind is the fundamental goal of physical fitness. It takes more than simply physical prowess to run a marathon or lift large objects; it takes strength, endurance, and flexibility to appreciate life fully.

Components of Physical Fitness

Cardiovascular endurance: is the capacity of the heart, lungs, and blood arteries to provide the working muscles with blood that is rich in oxygen while engaging in prolonged physical activity. Increasing cardiovascular endurance can lower the risk of cardiovascular illnesses and improve general stamina.

Muscular endurance: is the capacity of muscles to withstand prolonged, repeated contractions. It is essential for jobs demanding repetitive motions, like jogging, cycling, or swimming, as it enables extended performance of activities without exhaustion.

Flexibility: The range of mobility in one or more joints is referred to as flexibility. It is necessary to keep one's mobility intact, avoid injuries, and carry out tasks quickly and easily. Muscle stiffness can be decreased and flexibility can be enhanced by stretches.

Muscular Strength: Muscular strength is the maximum amount of force that a muscle or group of muscles can exert against resistance. It is essential for activities like lifting, pushing, and pulling heavy objects and can help prevent injuries and improve posture and stability.

Body Composition: Body composition refers to the proportion of fat, muscle, bone, and other tissues in the body. Achieving a healthy body composition, with a balance of lean muscle mass and minimal body fat, is essential for overall health and reducing the risk of obesity-related diseases.

The Value of Physical Fitness

Maintaining physical fitness is essential for fostering general health and well-being. The following are some main arguments in favor of physical fitness:

Better Health: Engaging in regular physical activity and exercise can help lower the chance of developing chronic illnesses including obesity, diabetes, and heart disease.

Enhanced Quality of Life: Being physically fit can improve energy levels, mood, and mental clarity, leading to a better overall quality of life.

Increased Longevity: Studies have shown that physically active individuals tend to live longer and enjoy a higher quality of life in their later years.

Better Functional Capacity: Physical fitness enables individuals to perform daily tasks more efficiently, reducing the risk of injury and enhancing independence.

Positive Body Image: By encouraging a healthy body composition and physical appearance, regular exercise can boost one's self-esteem and positive body image.

In conclusion, being physically healthy is about feeling good and experiencing life to the fullest, not only about looking nice. You may enhance your general quality of life and reap several health benefits by including regular exercise and physical activity in your regimen.

Benefits of Exercise and Physical Activity

Exercise and physical activity offer a wide range of benefits for both physical and mental health. In this chapter, we'll explore the various ways in which regular exercise can improve overall well-being.

Physical Health benefits

Frequent exercise improves physical health in a variety of ways, including:

Enhanced Cardiovascular Health: Exercise lowers the risk of high blood pressure, heart disease, and stroke by strengthening the heart and enhancing circulation.

Weight management: Exercise facilitates the burning of calories and the development of muscle, which makes it simpler to reach and maintain a healthy weight.

Enhanced Muscular Endurance and Strength: Exercises aimed at building muscle mass and tone facilitate daily tasks and lower the chance of injury.

Improved Bone Health: By helping to develop and maintain bone density, weight-bearing activities like walking, running, and resistance training lower the risk of osteoporosis and Increased Flexibility and Joint Health: Stretching exercises improve flexibility and range of motion, reducing the risk of injury and improving joint health.

Improved Immune Function: Regular physical activity boosts the immune system, making it easier to fight off infections and illnesses.

Reduced Risk of Chronic Diseases: Exercise can help prevent or manage a variety of chronic conditions, including type 2 diabetes, certain types of cancer, and metabolic syndrome.

Mental Health Benefits

Exercise not only improves physical health but also significantly improves mental health:

Decreased Stress and Anxiety: Exercise causes the brain's endorphins, which function as natural stress relievers, to be released, which lowers stress and anxiety levels.

Better Mood: Exercise increases the synthesis of neurotransmitters like dopamine and serotonin, which are linked to positive emotions and a sense of well-being.

Enhanced Cognitive Function: Research has demonstrated that exercise enhances memory, attention, and executive function. It may also lower the chance of cognitive loss associated with aging.

Improved Sleep: People who exercise regularly report feeling more rested and able to fall asleep more quickly. They also report that their sleep is longer and of higher quality.

Enhanced Confidence and Self-Esteem: Reaching fitness objectives and becoming more physically attractive via exercise can enhance confidence and self-esteem.

Social Connection: Taking part in team sports or group exercise programs can offer social support and opportunities for social engagement, which can help to lessen feelings of isolation and loneliness.

Long-Term Benefits of Regular Physical Activity

Regular physical activity has lifetime advantages that last a lifetime:

Increased Longevity: Research has linked regular exercise to a longer lifetime and a lower chance of passing away too soon.

Healthy Aging: Exercise lowers the risk of age-related impairments in mobility and cognitive function by preserving physical function and independence as people age.

Disease Prevention: Engaging in regular physical activity can help people age with better health and a higher quality of life by lowering their chance of developing chronic illnesses and disorders.

Improved Quality of Life: Engaging in regular exercise helps people stay healthy and energetic, which enables them to enjoy active, meaningful lives well into old age.

In conclusion, physical activity and exercise provide several advantages for mental and physical health, enhancing general well-being and raising quality of life. Your life can be more colorful, happier, and healthier if you exercise regularly.

Getting Started with Exercise

It's thrilling and powerful to start a journey of integrating exercise into your life. This chapter will cover the fundamentals of beginning an exercise regimen, such as goal-setting, planning a routine, and overcoming obstacles that often stand in the way of your success.

Setting Goals

In every fitness journey, the first step to success is setting clear and attainable goals. Here's how to make realistic fitness objectives:

Be Specific: Clearly define what you want to achieve with your exercise routine. Whether it's improving cardiovascular health, building strength, losing weight, or increasing flexibility, specificity will help you stay focused and motivated.

Make Them Measurable: Set quantifiable criteria to monitor your advancement toward your objectives. Establish goals for things like how many pounds you want to lift, how far you want to run, or how many days a week you want to work out.

Have Reasonable Expectations: Be reasonable about where you're starting from and how long it will take you to reach your objectives. Starting with smaller, more manageable milestones and working your way up is a better strategy to avoid setting too ambitious goals, which can cause dissatisfaction and fatigue.

Make Them Time-Bound: To foster a sense of urgency and accountability, assign yourself a deadline for finishing your goals. Having a timeline, no matter how long it is— one month, three months, or six—will keep you motivated and on track toward your goals.

Write Your Goals Down: Putting your objectives down on paper strengthens your will to see them through and gives them greater substance. Your goals should be in plain sight, such as in a diary or on a bulletin board, so you can see that every day your working towards your target.

Be Flexible: Remember that goals are not set in stone. It's okay to adjust your goals as needed based on your progress, preferences, and changing circumstances. The key is to stay adaptable and continue moving forward.

Making an Exercise Schedule

After you've determined your objectives, it's time to design an exercise program that suits your requirements and tastes. Here's how to create a fitness regimen that works:

Determine Your Present Fitness Level: To begin, determine your present level of fitness, taking into account your advantages, disadvantages, and any physical restrictions or health issues. This will support your goal-setting and exercise selection.

Choose Exercises and hobbies You Enjoy: Make sure your workouts and hobbies are things you look forward to performing. Whether you enjoy swimming, cycling, dancing, or hiking, including your favorite hobbies in your workout routine will help it become less of a hassle and more of an enjoyable and fulfilling experience.

Add Variety: To keep things fresh and avoid monotony, mix up your training routine with a range of exercises and activities. Incorporate cardiovascular, strength, and flexibility training, as well as balance and coordination-enhancing activities.

Establish a Timetable: Choose a regular exercise program and work it into your weekly calendar. Aim for two or more days of strength training activities in addition to at least 150 minutes of moderate-intensity aerobic activity or 75 minutes of vigorous-intensity aerobic activity each week.

Start Slowly: Whether you're brand-new to exercising or making a long-term return, begin with small steps and build up to greater intensity, longer exercises, and more frequent workouts. Pay attention to your body, take your time, make the necessary adjustments, and move forward at a comfortable pace for you.

Incorporate Rest and Recovery: Don't forget to incorporate days of rest into your exercise regimen so that your body has time to mend and recuperate. Rest is a vital part of any workout practice; ignore your body's signals and prioritize it. Overtraining can result in exhaustion, injuries, and burnout.

Monitor Your Progress: Keep a record of your workouts, your advancement toward your objectives, and any alterations to your level of fitness over time. This will assist you in staying inspired, pinpointing areas in need of development, and acknowledging your accomplishments as you go.

Overcoming Barriers to Exercise

You may have the best of intentions, but sometimes you run into roadblocks that throw off your fitness regimen. The following are some methods for getting beyond typical obstacles to exercise:

Lack of time: Schedule exercise into your daily schedule and treat it as important as any other appointment. Seek out opportunities to fit in little bursts of movement throughout the day, such going for a stroll during your lunch break or choosing to use the stairs rather than the elevator.

Lack of Motivation: Look for strategies to keep yourself inspired and motivated to work out, such as making modest, manageable objectives, rewarding yourself when you meet milestones, or finding a workout partner who will support and hold you accountable.

Fatigue or Low Energy: If you're feeling tired or low on energy, start with a lighter or less intense workout, such as a gentle walk or yoga session. Focus on activities that make you feel good and energized, and remember that even a little movement is better than none at all.

Fear of Injury: Start slowly and gradually increase the intensity and duration of your workouts to reduce the risk of injury. Pay attention to proper form and technique, listen to your body, and don't push yourself too hard too soon.

Lack of Access to Equipment or Facilities: You don't need fancy equipment or a gym membership to get a great workout. There are plenty of bodyweight exercises and activities you can do at home or outdoors with minimal equipment, such as walking, jogging, cycling, or using resistance bands.

Weather or Environmental Conditions: If weather or environmental conditions are preventing you from exercising outdoors, look for indoor alternatives such as walking or jogging on a treadmill, using a stationary bike or elliptical machine, or following along with a workout video or online fitness class.

Negative Self-Talk: Replace negative self-talk and self-doubt with positive affirmations and encouragement. Focus on your progress, celebrate your achievements, and goals.

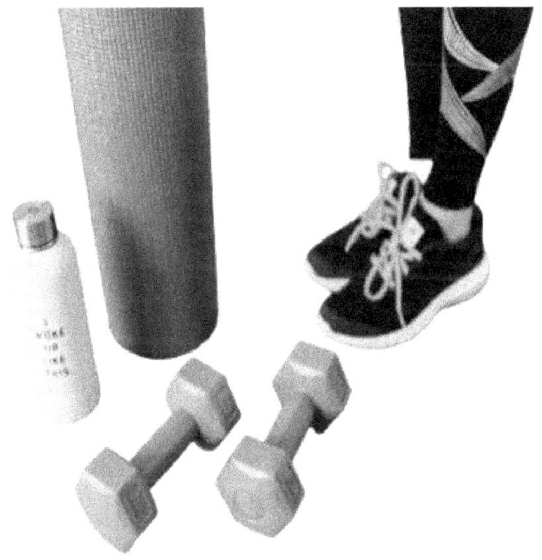

SECTION 1: FUNDAMENTAL EXERCISES

We'll look at the core components of exercise in this area, such as strength training, flexibility, and mobility exercises as well as cardiovascular exercises.

cardiovascular exercise

Aerobic exercise, sometimes referred to as cardiovascular exercise, is crucial for increasing endurance, burning calories, and heart health. Now let's explore the several facets of cardiovascular exercise:

Cardiovascular Exercise Types

There are numerous variations of cardiovascular exercise, and each has its advantages and difficulties. Walking is a low-impact activity that is suitable for most people. It increases muscle strength, burns calories, and strengthens the heart. Running and jogging are high-impact exercises that increase heart rate and boost endurance. They can be tailored to meet the needs of individuals with varying degrees of fitness.

Riding a bike: Riding a bike, whether indoors on a stationary cycle or outside on a road or path, is a great cardiovascular exercise that is easy on the joints.

Swimming: is a full-body, low-impact exercise that strengthens muscles, increases flexibility, and increases cardiovascular endurance.

Dancing: Whether you're into salsa or Zumba, dancing is an enjoyable and efficient technique to increase heart rate while enhancing balance and coordination.

Interval Training: This type of exercise maximizes cardiovascular benefits and calorie burn in a shorter length of time by alternating between periods of high-intensity activity and rest or low-intensity activity.

Cardiovascular Workouts for Beginners

For beginners, it's essential to start slowly and gradually increase intensity and duration. Here are some beginner-friendly cardiovascular workouts:

Brisk Walking: Aim for a brisk pace that elevates your heart rate but still allows you to carry on a conversation comfortably. Start with shorter walks and gradually increase distance and speed.

Cycling on Flat Terrain: Start with a leisurely bike ride on flat terrain to build cardiovascular endurance and get comfortable with the motion of cycling.

Swimming Laps: Start with a few laps at a comfortable pace, focusing on proper breathing and technique. Gradually increase the number of laps and intensity as your endurance improves.

Low-Impact Aerobic Classes: Join a low-impact aerobic class designed for beginners, such as water aerobics or beginner-friendly dance fitness classes.

Advanced Methods of Cardiovascular Exercise

Advanced training methods offer a more strenuous workout for individuals who want to push themselves and improve their cardiovascular fitness:

High-Intensity Interval Training (HIIT): HIIT workouts optimize calorie burn and cardiovascular effects in a shorter length of time by alternating between brief bursts of high-intensity activity and short rest periods.

Circuit Training: This full-body workout maintains a high heart rate by combining cardiovascular and strength-training activities performed quickly in succession with little rest in between sets.

Hill Training: Including hills or inclines in your aerobic exercises raises the intensity and develops the strength and power of your lower body.

Cross-Training: Mixing up your cardiovascular workouts with different activities, such as swimming, cycling, and running, prevents boredom, reduces the risk of overuse injuries, and improves overall fitness.

Strength Training

Strength training is crucial for building muscle mass, improving bone density, and boosting metabolism. Let's explore the fundamentals of strength training:

5.1 Benefits of Strength Training

Strength training offers numerous benefits for overall health and fitness:

Increased Muscle Mass: Strength training stimulates muscle growth, leading to increased muscle mass, strength, and endurance.

Improved Bone Density: Weight-bearing exercises like strength training help build and maintain bone density, reducing the risk of osteoporosis and fractures.

Enhanced Metabolism: Muscle tissue burns more calories at rest than fat tissue, so increasing muscle mass through strength training can boost metabolism and aid in weight management.

Better Joint Health: Strengthening the muscles around joints improves stability and reduces the risk of injury and joint pain.

Improved Functional Strength: Strength training exercises mimic real-life movements and activities, making everyday tasks easier and reducing the risk of falls and injuries.

Exercises for Strength Training Types

Exercises for strength training fall into several types, each focusing on a distinct set of muscles and movement patterns:

Compound Exercises: Compound exercises are a great way to improve general strength and muscular mass because they work with numerous joints and muscle groups. Pull-ups, bench presses, deadlifts, and squats are a few examples.

Isolation Exercises: Isolation exercises focus on certain muscle groups and help correct muscular imbalances and enhance muscle definition. Leg curls, tricep extensions, bicep curls, and calf lifts are a few examples.

Bodyweight Exercises: Bodyweight exercises are accessible and convenient for strength training because they use your body weight as resistance and require little equipment. Exercises like planks, squats, lunges, and push-ups are examples.

Free Weights: Free weights, such as dumbbells, barbells, and kettlebells, offer a versatile and effective way to build strength and muscle mass. They allow for a wide range of exercises and can be easily adjusted to accommodate different fitness levels.

Resistance Bands: Resistance bands provide variable resistance and are gentle on the joints, making them suitable for people of all fitness levels and abilities. They can be used to target specific muscle groups and add variety to your strength training routine.

Safely Increasing Strength and Muscle

Safety comes first when starting a strength training program. To safely increase your muscle and strength, abide by the following guidelines:

Start with Correct Form: Before advancing in weight or intensity, concentrate on perfecting the correct form and technique. Using proper form minimizes the chance of injury while simultaneously maximizing the efficiency of the activity.

Advance Gradually: As your strength and fitness level rise, start with lesser weights or resistance and progressively increase the weight, reps, or sets. Resist the urge to lift too much weight too quickly because this can cause injury or strain to the muscles.

Listen to Your Body: Pay attention to your body's signals and adjust your workout intensity or technique as needed. If you experience pain or discomfort during exercise, stop immediately and consult a fitness professional or healthcare provider.

Warm Up and Cool Down: Always start your strength training workout with a thorough warm-up to prepare your muscles and joints for exercise and end with a cool-down to promote recovery and flexibility.

Rest and Recovery: Allow your muscles time to rest and recover between strength training sessions. Aim for at least 48 hours of rest between workouts targeting the same muscle groups to prevent overtraining and promote muscle growth and repair.

Stay Hydrated and Nourished: Drink plenty of water before, during, and after your strength training workouts to stay hydrated. Fuel your body with a balanced diet rich in protein, carbohydrates, and healthy fats to support muscle growth and recovery.

Flexibility and Mobility

Flexibility and mobility are essential components of overall fitness and play a vital role in preventing injury and improving performance. Let's explore the importance of flexibility and mobility and how to improve them:

Importance of Flexibility

Flexibility refers to the range of motion in a joint or group of joints and is crucial for maintaining mobility and preventing injury. Here are some key benefits of flexibility training:

Increased Range of Motion: By increasing joint flexibility and range of motion, stretching exercises enable more fluid and effective movement.

Lower Risk of Injury: Sprains, sprains, and other injuries are less common in flexible muscles and joints.

Techniques for Stretching

Stretching exercises are a great way to increase your range of motion, flexibility, and general health. Here are some stretching methods you can attempt:

Static Stretching: Static stretching entails maintaining a stretch for a predetermined amount of time, typically 15 to 30 seconds. Stretches for the calf, shoulder, and hamstrings are a few examples.

Dynamic stretching: Usually performed as a part of a warm-up regimen, dynamic stretching entails carefully extending and contracting the body's range of motion. Walking lunges, leg swings, and arm circles are a few examples.

PNF Stretching: To increase flexibility, proprioceptive neuromuscular facilitation, or PNF stretching, entails tightening and relaxing the muscles surrounding a joint. This exercise is frequently performed with a resistance band or in pairs.

Yoga and Pilates: These forms of exercise include a range of stretches and strengthening movements to enhance flexibility, balance, and strength of the core. Additionally, these mind-body techniques aid in stress reduction and relaxation.

Pilates and Yoga to Increase Flexibility

Popular mind-body exercises that emphasize strength, flexibility, and relaxation are yoga and pilates. They can increase mobility and flexibility in the following ways:

Yoga: Yoga consists of a sequence of positions, or asanas, that strengthen and stretch the body while encouraging awareness and relaxation. Frequent yoga practice enhances posture, flexibility, and balance, which facilitates fluid and graceful movement.

Pilates: Using a series of carefully timed movements, either on a mat or with specialized equipment, Pilates focuses on core strength, stability, and body awareness. Pilates workouts enhance overall mobility and function by promoting better posture, muscle tone, and flexibility.

You may develop a strong, resilient, and healthy body by including aerobic activity, strength training, and mobility and flexibility exercises in your fitness regimen. These workout fundamentals will put you on the right track to success whether you're a novice trying to get started or an expert looking to increase your level of fitness.

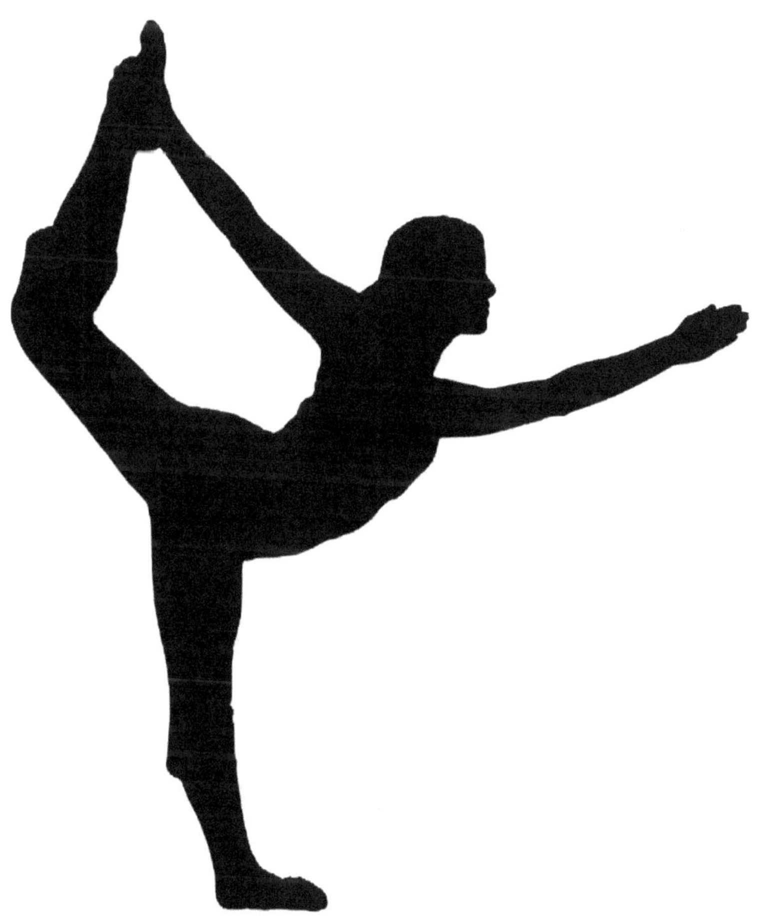

SECTION 2: PHYSICAL ACTIVITIES

This section will cover a variety of topics related to integrating physical activity into your daily life, such as family-friendly exercise activities, workplace wellness initiatives, and active transportation. We'll also explore sports and outdoor activity, as well as mind-body practices that support general well-being, stress management, and mindfulness.

Integrating Exercise into Everyday Life

Exercise doesn't have to be limited to set workout times or gym memberships. You can get the health advantages of physical activity while going about your regular business if you incorporate movement into your routine.

Active Transportation

Using human-powered means of transportation—like cycling, walking, or public transportation—instead of relying on automobiles is known as active transportation.

The following are some ideas for integrating active transportation into your everyday schedule:

Walking or Cycling to Work: Rather than driving or using public transportation, if at all possible, think about walking or cycling to work. This encourages environmental sustainability and lowers carbon emissions in addition to offering a chance for physical activity.

Choosing the steps: Whenever feasible, choose the steps over the elevator. Stair climbing is a great strategy to increase heart rate and build muscle in your lower body.

strolling Meetings: Suggest having strolling meetings with coworkers rather than seated in a conference room. Talking and strolling together not only encourages exercise but also increases productivity and creativity.

Workplace Wellness Strategies

Many people spend a significant portion of their day at work, making it an ideal opportunity to incorporate physical activity into the workday. Here are some workplace wellness strategies to consider:

Desk Exercises: Incorporate short exercise breaks into your workday by doing desk exercises like seated leg lifts, chair squats, or shoulder stretches.

Standing Desks: Consider using a standing desk or adjustable workstation that allows you to alternate between sitting and standing throughout the day. Standing desks can help reduce sedentary behavior and alleviate back pain.

Fitness Challenges: Organize workplace fitness challenges or wellness programs to encourage employees to stay active and healthy. This could include step challenges, fitness classes, or healthy eating initiatives.

Family-Friendly Exercise Programs

Engaging in physical activities with close companions enhances its enjoyment. Try these family-friendly exercise activities:

Family Bike Rides or Walks: Make the most of your time together by taking your family on bike rides or walks through the neighborhood or nearby park.

Backyard Games: Set up family-friendly backyard activities like soccer, frisbee, and tag.

Fitness class for kids: Enroll kids in age-appropriate sports leagues or fitness courses to expose them to a range of physical activities and foster a lifetime love of exercise.

Sports and Outdoor Recreation

Sports and outdoor activities provide a chance to interact with nature, push your physical limits, and socialize with others. Check out these well-liked outdoor pursuits:

Trail Running and Hiking

A terrific way to explore nature and work out your whole body is to go hiking or trail running. Trail running and hiking have mental and physical benefits, whether you're jogging through beautiful scenery, climbing mountains, or navigating forest routes.

Cycling and Bicycling

People of all ages and fitness levels can enjoy the various sports of cycling and biking. Cycling offers a great cardiovascular workout and a chance to get outside and enjoy nature, whether you're riding through urban areas, rural roads, or steep mountain paths.

Group Activities and Team Sports

In addition to the physical advantages, team sports and group activities promote social connection, camaraderie, and a sense of belonging. There is something for everyone to enjoy, whether they like group activities like rock climbing, kayaking, or paddleboarding, or team sports like basketball, volleyball, or soccer.

Mind-Body Practices

The goal of mind-body exercises is to integrate the mind and body to facilitate overall well-being, stress reduction, and relaxation. These are a few well-liked mind-body exercises to explore:

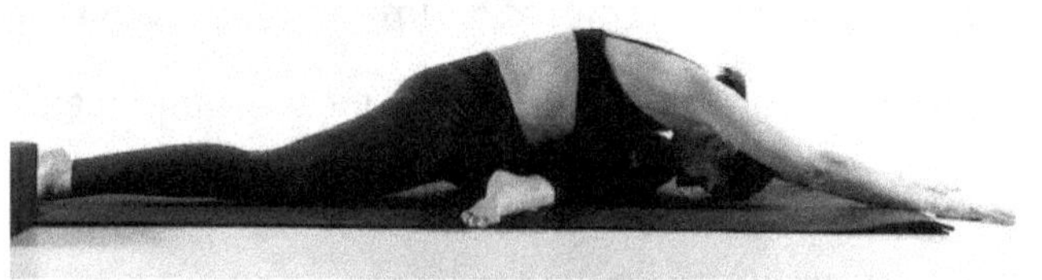

Yoga for Mindfulness and Stress Reduction

Yoga combines physical postures, breathwork, and meditation to promote relaxation, flexibility, and inner peace. Whether you're practicing gentle hatha yoga, dynamic vinyasa flow, or restorative yin yoga, yoga provides a holistic approach to health and wellness.

Pilates for Core Strength and Stability

Pilates focuses on strengthening the core muscles, improving posture, and enhancing body awareness and alignment. Through a series of controlled movements performed on a mat or using specialized equipment, Pilates builds core strength, stability, and flexibility for improved overall function and movement.

Tai Chi and Qigong for Balance and Harmony

Tai Chi and Qigong are ancient Chinese practices that combine gentle movements, deep breathing, and mindfulness to promote balance, harmony, and vitality. Whether you're practicing the slow, flowing movements of Tai Chi or the dynamic energy exercises of Qigong, these mind-body practices cultivate relaxation, reduce stress, and improve physical and mental well-being.

Incorporating physical activity into your daily life, enjoying outdoor recreation and sports, and exploring mind-body activities are excellent ways to stay active, healthy, and engaged. Whether you're seeking adventure, relaxation, or simply looking to improve your overall well-being, there's a physical activity or sport to suit your interests and lifestyle.

SECTION 3: PILATES PRACTICES

We will explore the realm of Pilates in this section. Pilates is a body-aware workout method that emphasizes flexibility, strength in the core, and total body awareness.

Introduction to Pilates

Joseph Pilates created the mind-body exercise method known as Pilates in the early 1900s. With an emphasis on deliberate movements and breath awareness, it highlights core strength, flexibility, and good alignment. Let's examine the background, tenets, and application of Pilates:

Background and Origins of Pilates

During World War I, Joseph Pilates created the Pilates method in the 1920s to help wounded troops heal. With a background in gymnastics, yoga, and martial arts, Pilates developed a set of exercises that strengthen the body and encourage proper alignment and balance. Since then, Pilates has developed into a well-liked exercise regimen that individuals of all ages and physical levels have adopted.

Principles of Pilates Practice

The Pilates method is guided by several key principles that inform the execution of exercises and the overall practice:

Breath: Proper breathing is essential in Pilates, with an emphasis on deep, diaphragmatic breathing to facilitate movement, oxygenation, and relaxation.

Concentration: Pilates requires focused attention and concentration on each movement, encouraging mindfulness and body awareness.

Control: Exercises are performed with precision and control, emphasizing quality of movement over quantity.

Centering: Pilates focuses on strengthening the core muscles, often referred to as the "powerhouse," which includes the muscles of the abdomen, lower back, hips, and buttocks.

Precision: Exercises are performed with attention to alignment, form, and muscle engagement, ensuring optimal effectiveness and safety.

Flow: Pilates exercises are typically performed in a flowing, continuous manner, with smooth transitions between movements to promote fluidity and grace.

Integration: Pilates seeks to integrate mind, body, and breath, fostering a holistic approach to health and fitness.

Equipment and Mat Pilates

Pilates can be performed on a basic mat with little equipment or with sophisticated tools like the chair, Cadillac, and reformer. Pilates on equipment and mat Pilates each have special advantages and difficulties that let practitioners customize their practice to meet their requirements and objectives.

Pilates Exercises to Build Core Stability

The foundation of Pilates practice is core strength, with movements aimed at stabilizing and strengthening the muscles of the lower back, pelvis, and abdomen. Let's look at some Pilates poses that target the core:

Mat Pilates Core Workouts

Mat Pilates exercises can be performed on a padded mat with no additional equipment, making them accessible and convenient for home practice. Here are some core-strengthening Pilates exercises you can try:

The Hundred: A classic Pilates exercise that targets the abdominal muscles and promotes core stability and endurance.

Roll-Up: A dynamic exercise that strengthens the abdominals and improves spinal mobility and flexibility.

Plank Variations: Plank exercises, such as forearm plank and side plank, engage the entire core and promote strength, stability, and alignment.

Leg Circles: Leg circle exercises challenge the core muscles while improving hip mobility and flexibility.

Reformer Exercises for Core Stability

The Pilates reformer is a versatile piece of equipment that provides resistance and support for a wide range of exercises. Here are some core-strengthening Pilates reformer exercises:

Footwork: Footwork exercises on the reformer target the core muscles while improving leg strength and alignment.

Long Stretch Series: The long stretch series on the reformer challenges core stability and control while promoting flexibility and balance.

Short Box Series: The short box series on the reformer includes exercises such as the stomach massage and twist, which target the abdominals and obliques while improving spinal mobility.

Advanced Pilates Techniques for Abdominal Strength

For those looking to take their core strength to the next level, advanced Pilates techniques offer a more challenging workout:

Teaser: The teaser is an advanced Pilates exercise that requires core strength, stability, and control to lift the body into a V-shape position while balancing on the sit bones.

Swan Dive: The swan dive exercise strengthens the entire posterior chain while promoting spinal extension and mobility.

Control Balance: The control balance exercise challenges core stability and control while balancing on the reformer carriage with the legs extended and the upper body lifted.

Pilates for Flexibility and Posture

In addition to core strength, Pilates emphasizes flexibility and proper alignment, promoting better posture and overall body awareness. Let's explore how Pilates can improve flexibility and posture:

Stretching and Lengthening with Pilates

Pilates incorporates stretching and lengthening exercises to improve flexibility and range of motion in the muscles and joints. Here are some Pilates exercises that promote flexibility:

The Saw: The saw exercise stretches the muscles of the spine, shoulders, and hamstrings while promoting spinal rotation and flexibility.

The Swan: The swan exercise stretches the muscles of the chest, abdomen, and hip flexors while promoting spinal extension and mobility.

Mermaid Stretch: The mermaid stretch targets the muscles of the side body and promotes lateral flexion and spinal mobility.

Improving Posture and Alignment

Pilates exercises are designed to promote proper alignment and posture by strengthening the muscles that support the spine and pelvis. Here are some Pilates exercises that improve posture:

The Shoulder Bridge: The shoulder bridge exercise strengthens the muscles of the back, buttocks, and hamstrings while promoting spinal alignment and stability.

The Swan Dive: The swan dive exercise strengthens the muscles of the upper back and shoulders while promoting extension and alignment of the spine.

The Chest Expansion: The chest expansion exercise targets the muscles of the chest, shoulders, and upper back, helping to counteract the effects of slouching and rounded shoulders.

Pilates for Spinal Health and Mobility

Pilates exercises are beneficial for spinal health and mobility, helping to alleviate stiffness and improve range of motion in the spine. Here are some Pilates exercises that promote spinal health:

Spinal Twist: The spinal twist exercise promotes spinal rotation and mobility while stretching the muscles of the spine and torso.

The Cat-Cow Stretch: The cat-cow stretch helps to mobilize the spine and improve flexibility and range of motion in the back and hips.

The Roll-Up: The roll-up exercise strengthens the muscles of the spine and torso

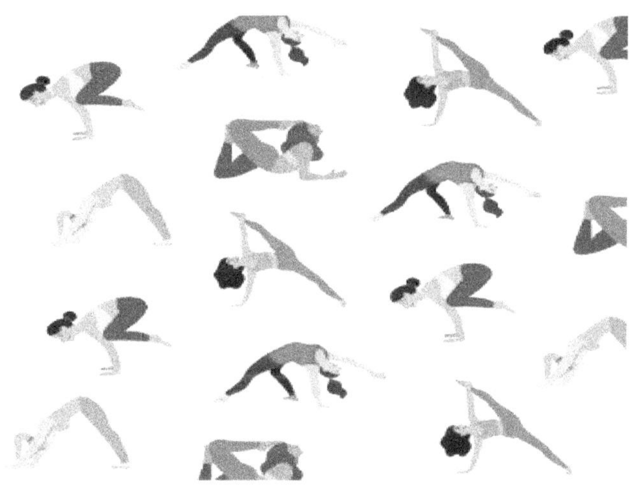

30-Day Exercise and Pilates Challenge

Introducing the "30-Day Exercise and Pilates Challenge," an amazing journey that will assist you in toning, strengthening, and revitalizing both your body and mind. You'll start a monthly regimen of Pilates exercises and everyday workouts that will increase your flexibility, vigor, and general well-being. Prepare to dedicate yourself to 30 days of activity, development, and self-exploration!

Week 1: Building Foundations

Day 1: Introduction to the Challenge

- Welcome to the 30-day exercise and Pilates challenge! Take some time to familiarize yourself with the challenge goals, guidelines, and schedule. Set your intentions for the next 30 days and commit to prioritizing your health and well-being.

Day 2: **Full-Body Stretching Routine**

- Start your challenge with a gentle full-body stretching routine to awaken your muscles and increase flexibility. Focus on deep breathing and mindful movement as you stretch each major muscle group, including the neck, shoulders, back, hips, and legs.

Day 3: **Basic Pilates Mat Workout**

- Begin your Pilates journey with a basic mat workout that introduces you to fundamental Pilates exercises. Focus on proper alignment, control, and breath as you perform exercises such as the Hundred, Roll-Up, Single Leg Stretch, and Bridge.

Day 4: **Lower Body Focus: Squats and Lunges**

- Strengthen and tone your lower body with a focus on squats and lunges. These compound exercises target the muscles of the legs, hips, and glutes while also engaging the core for stability. Perform variations such as sumo squats, reverse lunges, and side lunges to challenge different muscle groups.

Day 5 Upper Body Strength: Push-Ups and Planks

- Build upper body strength and stability with a series of push-up and plank variations. These bodyweight exercises target the chest, shoulders, triceps, and core muscles. Experiment with different hand placements and modifications to suit your fitness level.

Day 6: Core Challenge: Hundred and Roll-Up

- Challenge your core with the classic Pilates Hundred exercise, which involves pumping your arms while engaging your abdominals. Follow it up with the Roll-Up, a dynamic exercise that strengthens the entire core and improves spinal mobility. Focus on controlled movement and precision.

Day 7: Rest and Recovery Day

- Take a well-deserved rest day to allow your body to recover and rejuvenate. Use this time to prioritize self-care activities such as gentle stretching, foam rolling, meditation, or a leisurely walk. Listen to your body and honor its need for rest and relaxation.

Week 2: Deepening Your Practice

Day 8: Dynamic Warm-Up and Mobility Exercises

- Begin your day with a dynamic warm-up routine that includes dynamic stretches and mobility exercises to prepare your body for movement. Focus on movements that target the major joints and muscles, such as arm circles, leg swings, hip circles, and torso twists.

Day 9: Pilates Ring (Magic Circle) Routine

- Incorporate the Pilates ring (also known as the magic circle) into your workout for added resistance and muscle engagement. Perform a series of Pilates exercises using the ring to target the arms, legs, and core muscles. Focus on maintaining proper form and controlled movements throughout.

Day 10: Pilates Reformer Series: Leg Work

- Explore leg-focused Pilates exercises inspired by the movements performed on the Pilates reformer. Use a mat or stability ball to mimic the resistance provided by the reformer machine. Perform exercises such as leg circles, leg presses, and leg lifts to strengthen and tone the lower body.

Day 11: Pilates Reformer Series: Arm Work

- Continue your Pilates journey with a series of arm-focused exercises inspired by the Pilates reformer. Use resistance bands or light dumbbells to simulate the resistance provided by the reformer springs. Perform exercises such as arm circles, bicep curls, triceps presses, and shoulder presses to sculpt and tone the arms.

Day 12: Balance and Stability: Single-Leg Exercises

- Challenge your balance and stability with a series of single-leg exercises that target the lower body and core muscles. Perform exercises such as single-leg squats, single-leg deadlifts, and single-leg balances to improve balance, coordination, and proprioception.

Day 13: Flexibility Focus: Hamstring and Hip Flexor Stretches

- Focus on improving flexibility and mobility in the hamstrings and hip flexors with a series of dynamic and static stretches. Perform stretches such as standing hamstring stretches, seated hip flexor stretches, and supine hamstring stretches to increase flexibility and reduce tightness in these muscle groups.

Day 14: Active Recovery Day: Gentle Yoga Flow

- Take a break from intense exercise and enjoy a gentle yoga flow designed to promote relaxation and recovery. Focus on slow, flowing movements and deep breathing as you move through a sequence of yoga poses that stretch and release tension from the body. Allow yourself to unwind and rejuvenate both physically and mentally.

Top of Form

Week 3: Strengthen and Energize

Day 15: High-Intensity Interval Training (HIIT) Workout

- Get your heart pumping with a high-intensity interval training (HIIT) workout that alternates between bursts of intense exercise and short periods of rest. Incorporate exercises such as burpees, jumping jacks, mountain climbers, and squat jumps to elevate your heart rate and torch calories.

Day 16: Cardio Pilates Fusion: Dance Inspired Moves

- Combine the benefits of cardio and Pilates with a fun and dynamic workout inspired by dance moves.

Incorporate rhythmic movements, flowing transitions, and Pilates principles to sculpt and tone your body while improving cardiovascular fitness and coordination.

Day 17: Full-Body Sculpting: Resistance Band Exercises

- Grab a resistance band and sculpt your entire body with a series of resistance band exercises. Target major muscle groups including the arms, shoulders, chest, back, legs, and glutes with exercises such as bicep curls, shoulder presses, rows, squats, and lunges.

Day 18: Pilates Ball (Exercise Ball) Routine

- Challenge your stability and core strength with a Pilates ball (exercise ball) routine. Perform a series of exercises using the ball to engage the core, improve balance, and enhance flexibility. Focus on controlled movements and proper form to maximize effectiveness.

Day 19: Power Yoga Flow: Strength and Flexibility

- Energize your body and mind with a power yoga flow that combines strength-building poses with flowing movements and deep stretches. Focus on linking breath with movement as you move through a dynamic sequence designed to build strength, flexibility, and endurance.

Day 20: Core Burnout: Advanced Pilates Techniques

- Take your core strength to the next level with a challenging Pilates workout that targets the deep abdominal muscles. Incorporate advanced Pilates techniques such as the teaser, scissors, and crisscross to sculpt and define your core.

Day 21: Active Rest Day: Walking or Gentle Hike

- Enjoy an active rest day by engaging in low-impact exercise such as walking or hiking. Take advantage of the outdoors and explore nature while giving your body a break from intense workouts. Focus on moving at a comfortable pace and enjoying the scenery.

Week 4: Integration and Reflection

Day 22: Pilates for Posture: Back Strengthening Exercises

- Focus on improving posture and strengthening the muscles of the back with a series of Pilates exercises. Target areas such as the upper back, lower back, and shoulders to promote proper alignment and reduce the risk of back pain.

Day 23: Pilates Flow for Mindfulness and Relaxation

- Take time to unwind and de-stress with a gentle Pilates flow focused on mindfulness and relaxation. Connect with your breath and move through a series of slow, fluid movements designed to release tension and promote a sense of calm and well-being.

Day 24: Endurance Challenge: Long-Duration Cardio

- Push your endurance to the limit with a long-duration cardio workout. Choose your favorite cardiovascular activity such as running, cycling, swimming, or hiking, and aim to maintain a steady pace for an extended period of time to build stamina and cardiovascular fitness.

Day 25: Pilates for Balance: Stability Ball Exercises

- Improve balance and stability with a series of Pilates exercises using a stability ball. Focus on engaging the core and stabilizing muscles as you perform exercises such as ball bridges, ball squats, and ball rollouts to challenge your balance and coordination.

Day 26: Yin Yoga: Deep Stretching and Relaxation

- Indulge in a deep stretching and relaxation session with Yin yoga. Hold passive stretches for an extended period of time to target the connective tissues and release tension from the body. Focus on surrendering to the poses and allowing yourself to fully relax and let go.

Day 27: Pilates Fusion: Barre Inspired Workout

- Combine elements of Pilates and barre with a fusion workout that targets the entire body. Incorporate small, controlled movements and isometric holds to sculpt and tone muscles while improving strength, flexibility, and posture.

Day 28: Reflection Day: Journaling and Goal Setting

- Take time to reflect on your journey over the past four weeks. Journal about your progress, achievements, and challenges, and take stock of how far you've come. Set new goals and intentions for the future, and reaffirm your commitment to your health and well-being.

Week 5: Celebration and Continuation

Day 29: **Full-Body Pilates Party: Dance and Movement**

- Celebrate your achievements with a full-body Pilates party featuring dance-inspired movements and dynamic exercises. Let loose, have fun, and enjoy the feeling of strength and vitality in your body as you move to the beat.

Day 30: **Final Challenge: Putting It All Together**

- Challenge yourself with a final workout that incorporates elements from each week of the challenge. Combine cardio, strength, flexibility, and mindfulness exercises to create a comprehensive full-body workout that showcases your progress and achievements.

Celebration and Reflection

- Congratulations on completing the 30-day exercise and Pilates challenge! Take time to celebrate your accomplishments and reflect on the positive changes you've experienced in your body and mind. Use this day to celebrate your journey and set intentions for continued growth and well-being.

In summary

Exercise, physical fitness, and mindful movement are all essential components of the path to improved health and wellness. As we get to the end of this extensive book, it's critical to understand that pursuing long-term fitness and wellness involves adopting a holistic lifestyle that is oriented around self-care, exercise, and mindfulness rather than just reaching a certain goal.

13.1 Establishing Long-Term Workout Routines

Developing enduring workout routines is essential to preserving long-term health and fitness. When it comes to your attitude to physical activity, give consistency, enjoyment, and balance top priority instead of only short-term goals. Make time for the things that you truly enjoy doing on a regular basis. Set attainable objectives, pay attention to your body, and be adaptable while changing up your workout routine to fit your lifestyle and needs.

Finding Joy and Satisfaction in Movement

Movement should be a source of joy and satisfaction, not a chore or obligation. Embrace a mindset of exploration and curiosity, and be open to trying new activities and experiences. Whether it's dancing, hiking, practicing yoga, or engaging in team sports, find activities that bring you happiness and fulfillment. Cultivate gratitude for your body's capabilities and celebrate the progress and achievements, no matter how small.

Exploration and Ongoing Education

The quest for health and fitness is a lifetime endeavor that presents countless chances for development and education. Continue to learn about various facets of physical fitness, exercise, and holistic well-being. Remain inquisitive and receptive. Investigate novel movement modalities, methods, and strategies, and look for chances for both professional and personal growth. Always keep in mind that every action you do to better yourself is an important investment in your general well-being.

www.ingramcontent.com/pod-product-compliance
Lightning Source LLC
Chambersburg PA
CBHW050850260726
48660CB00006B/2544